MW01286314

Table of Contents

INTRODUCTION

SIBO has gotten a lot of press recently, most likely due to its increasing prevalence in recent years. SIBO stands for small intestinal bacterial overgrowth, and is defined as a chronic infection of the small intestine. The most common symptoms of SIBO are very similar to that of IBS - namely gas, bloating, diarrhea, constipation, leaky gut, fructose malabsorption and excessive fermentation of certain carbohydrates called FODMAPs. If you're suffering from SIBO you may also experience eczema, joint pain, headaches, asthma, depression, autoimmune disorders and a multitude of food sensitivities. According to research by Dr. Mark Pimental, 84% of people with IBS have bacterial overgrowth in their small intestine which could suggest that most people who complain of IBS symptoms also have SIBO. (Most IBS patients are FODMAP intolerant, but while consuming FODMAPs exacerbates symptoms, it doesn't actually cause IBS.)Because it can be so difficult to treat it requires a combination of specific diet, special treatment (including antibiotics and/or herbal therapies) and certain herbs to help boost intestinal movement (AKA prokinetics).

All of these need to be balanced while trying to find and treat the CAUSE of SIBO. If you don't address the cause of the SIBO, then it is likely to come right back - even after treatment! If you've been recently diagnosed with SIBO or you're wondering what types of food you can/should eat then this is the Book for you. Did I mention that I also suffered from SIBO and used this exact treatment plan to heal myself? Because I've been through this and have experienced the symptoms I've gone through great lengths to make this a VERY comprehensive guide...

We are going to dive into ALL of the following in detail:

- What you should and shouldn't be eating
- All the symptoms of SIBO and what to do if you think you have it
- The connection between SIBO and Hypothyroidism that you don't want to miss
- The Diet I use on my patients and have had significant success with

- How to treat SIBO (Using antibiotics and/or herbal therapies)

What Is SIBO

SIBO is the acronym for "small intestinal bacterial overgrowth," defined as excessive bacteria in the small intestine, or small bowel. While bacteria naturally occurs throughout the digestive tract, in a healthy system, the small intestine has relatively low levels of bacteria; it's supposed to be at highest concentrations in the colon.

The small intestine is the longest section of the digestive tract. This is where the food intermingles with digestive juices, and the nutrients are absorbed into the bloodstream. If SIBO is indicated, malabsorption of nutrients, particularly fat-soluble vitamins and iron, can quickly become a problem.

When in proper balance, the bacteria in the colon helps digest foods and the body absorb essential nutrients.

However, when bacteria invades and takes over the small intestine, it can lead to poor nutrient absorption, symptoms commonly associated with IBS, and may even lead to damage of the stomach lining.

When you have SIBO, as food passes through the small intestine, the bacterial overgrowth interferes with the healthy digestive and absorption process. The bacterium associated with SIBO actually consumes some of the foods and nutrients, leading to unpleasant SIBO symptoms, including gas, bloating and pain.

Even when treating small intestinal bacterial overgrowth with antibiotics, relapse rate is high. This is a chronic condition that can be cured, but it takes patience, perseverance and a change in diet. In fact, SIBO treatment includes a healing diet, and some foods should be avoided until the gut flora is back in balance.

SIBO Symptoms

The indications of SIBO mirror the symptoms of other gastrointestinal disorders, including IBS. According to a study published in the World Journal of Gastroenterology, there's good reason for the similar symptoms there's a definite association between IBS and SIBO. Researchers suggest that physicians give consideration of excluding SIBO before giving a definitive diagnosis of IBS.

Common symptoms of SIBO and IBS include:

- Nausea
- Bloating
- Vomiting
- Diarrhea
- Malnutrition
- Weight loss
- Joint pain
- Fatigue
- Rashes
- Acne
- Eczema
- Asthma
- Depression
- Rosacea

Causes and Risk Factors of SIBO

There are a number of underlying conditions believed to contribute to small intestine bacterial overgrowth. These include aging, dysmotility (when muscles in the digestive system don't work properly), chronic pancreatitis, diabetes, diverticulosis, a structural defect in the small intestine, injury, fistula, intestinal lymphoma and scleroderma.

The use of certain medications, including immunosuppressant medications, proton pump inhibitors, immune system disorders, recent abdominal surgery and celiac disease are also associated with an increased risk for developing SIBO. Celiac disease can be of particular concern as it disturbs gut motility leading to improper small intestine functioning.

According to a study published in the American Journal of Gastroenterology, 66 percent of patients with celiac disease who maintained a strict gluten-free diet tested positive for bacterial overgrowth. In this study, patients were treated individually with a combination of antibiotics, prescription medications for worms and parasites, and a change in diet. All patients reported their symptoms were abated after SIBO treatment.

Another underlying cause of SIBO symptoms is blind loop syndrome. This occurs when the small intestine actually forms a loop, causing food to bypass parts of the digestive tract. This causes food to move more slowly through the system, and the result is a breeding ground for bacteria.

Metabolic disorders, including type 2 diabetes that's not properly controlled, are believed to lead or contribute to certain gastrointestinal disorders. In fact, a study published in Diabetes & Metabolism indicates that SIBO was present in 43 percent of diabetics with chronic diabetes.

Aging is another risk factor for developing small intestine bacterial overgrowth. As we age, the digestive tract slows down. It's generally accepted that non-hospitalized adults over the age of 61 have a 15 percent prevalence rate of SIBO, in contrast with just under 6 percent in individuals 24 to 59 years old. A study published in the Journal of the

American Geriatric Society also found that over 30 percent of disabled older adults have SIBO.

Rosacea, a skin condition that causes redness and rashes on the face, is also associated with SIBO symptoms. Researchers from the Department of Internal Medicine at the University of Genoa in Italy found that rosacea patients have a significantly higher prevalence rate of SIBO.

For those who suffer with rosacea, there's good news — this study also indicates "an almost complete regression of their cutaneous lesions and maintained this excellent result for at least 9 months" after the eradication of SIBO.

As you can see, small intestinal bacterial overgrowth is linked, caused or associated with a wide array of conditions. Even those not thought to be related to the gastrointestinal tract seem to correlate with SIBO symptoms.

Breath Testing for SIBO

In order to diagnose SIBO, doctors use a hydrogen breath test to measure the amount of gas produced by the bacteria in the small intestine. The test measures the amount of hydrogen and methane in your body. This works because the only way the human body produces these gases is through the output of bacteria. A solution containing one of the following sugars is used to complete the breath test:

- Lactulose
- Glucose
- Xylose

First the patient participates in a special diet for two days prior to the test. Then the patient drinks a solution containing one of the sugars listed above, which feeds the bacteria. The breath test measures how much hydrogen and methane has been produced by the bacteria as a result. These results allow your health care professional to determine if you are experiencing SIBO.

Complications Associated with SIBO

SIBO, left untreated, can cause potentially serious health complications. It's vital to get rid of the bacterial overgrowth as soon as possible. Bacteria overgrowth in the small intestine can lead to malnutrition, one of the biggest concerns with SIBO. Essential nutrients, protein, carbohydrates and fats aren't properly absorbed, causing deficiencies, including iron deficiency, vitamin B12 deficiency, calcium deficiency and deficiencies in the fat-soluble vitamins vitamin A deficiency, vitamin D deficiency, vitamin E deficiency and vitamin K deficiency.

These deficiencies can lead to symptoms, including weakness, fatigue, confusion and damage to the central nervous symptom.

Vitamin B12 deficiency is more common than most people believe. There are a number of factors that can lead to deficiency, besides SIBO. Vegetarians and vegans are at particular risk, as are individuals who have inadequate stomach acid or take medications that suppress stomach acid such as proton pump inhibitors, H2 blockers and other antacids.

As noted above, these commonly prescribed medications are linked to SIBO.

According to Harvard Medical School, the symptoms of vitamin B12 deficiency can appear gradually or very rapidly. Symptoms may include numbness or tingling in extremities, anemia, jaundice, decline in cognitive function, memory loss, fatigue, weakness, and even paranoia or hallucinations.

In a report in the British Journal of Haematology, researchers indicate that megaloblastic anemia, a blood disorder that causes the loss of red blood cells, is directly related to bacterial overgrowth in the small intestine. This is due to the malabsorption of vitamin B12.

If you have SIBO or a vitamin B12 deficiency, it's imperative to catch megaloblastic anemia quickly; prolonged vitamin B12 deficiency can lead to permanent nerve damage. If you experience any of these symptoms of vitamin B12 deficiency, in addition to any of the common SIBO symptoms mentioned above, take charge of your health, and get started ridding your body of small intestinal bacteria.

Treating SIBO

Small intestinal bacterial overgrowth is most often treated with antibiotics such as rifaximin (brand name Xifaxan). This helps reduce the problem bacteria but also kills off the healthy bacteria necessary for proper digestive functioning. For some patients with SIBO caused by blind loop syndrome, long-term antibiotic courses may be required. Even with antibiotics, SIBO is difficult to treat. In fact, a study published in the American Journal of Gastroenterology, researchers concluded SIBO patients treated with antibiotics have a high recurrence rate and that gastrointestinal symptoms increased during the recurrences.

The good news is that researchers have found that herbal remedies are as effective as three courses of antibiotic therapy in patients who don't respond well to rifaximin. This study mentions a variety of herbal remedies but doesn't include dosing or further details. Oregano oil, berberine extract, wormwood oil, lemon balm oil and Indian barberry root extract are all mentioned in the study. So how do you treat SIBO and SIBO symptoms? First, it's important to identify if there's an underlying cause. The next step is to start reversing the nutritional deficiencies. A healthy diet, nutritional supplements and lifestyle changes are necessary to get the body back in balance.

My first recommendation to overcome SIBO is to consume smaller amounts of food during meals. Spread your meals out at 5–6 smaller portions per day rather than 3 larger meals. Eating smaller meals allows you to digest foods more quickly, which is crucial to overcoming SIBO. Overeating is one of the worst things for SIBO because it causes food to sit longer in the stomach and can also damage gastric juice production. Low stomach acid production is one of the main contributing factors of SIBO because stomach acid kills off bacteria in your upper GI regions.

Next, one of the key things you can do today to help get rid of small intestinal bacterial overgrowth is to start probiotic supplements and eat probiotic-rich foods immediately. A pilot study from researchers at the Center for Medical Education and Clinical Research in Buenos Aires, Argentina, found probiotics have a higher efficacy rate than metronidazole for individuals with SIBO.

In this study, Lactobacillus casei, Lactobacillus plantarum, Streptococcus faecalis and Bifidobacterium brevis were administered for five days to half of the study group, while the other half of the study group received antibiotics for five days. All participants ate the same diet, which limited consumption of dairy products, legumes, leafy green vegetables and alcohol.

The results? An astounding 82 percent of the group receiving probiotics reported clinical improvement, while only 52 percent of the group receiving antibiotics reported clinical improvement.

In addition to probiotics and combatting nutrient deficiencies, it's important to change your diet.

Supplements for SIBO

These are the supplements that most commonly come up for SIBO symptoms and treatment and overcoming the nutritional deficiencies caused by SIBO. Follow RDA levels for each, as supplement research for overcoming SIBO is in its infancy.

- Vitamin B12
- Vitamin D
- Vitamin K
- Probiotics
- Digestive Enzymes
- Iron
- Zinc

Essential Oils for SIBO

In addition to dietary changes and supplements, the use of essential oils has been shown to be helpful for people with

SIBO symptoms. In a case report published in the Alternative Medicine Review, peppermint oil is shown to provide relief from certain gastrointestinal symptoms, including IBS and others.

This report highlighted the use of enteric-coated peppermint oil in the treatment of IBS, chronic fatigue syndrome and fibromyalgia. A single patient with SIBO reported marked improvement with peppermint oil, and researchers indicated that further investigation is needed.

Other essential oils that may be beneficial when treating SIBO symptoms include oregano oil, tarragon oil, frankincense oil, clove oil and others. Use only high-quality, food-grade essential oils. A drop or two in a glass of water prior to a meal can help reduce boating and gas, as well as other symptoms of digestive upset.

Lifestyle Changes for SIBO

A few lifestyle changes may also be helpful in healing your digestive system and getting rid of SIBO symptoms. In both phase 1 and phase 2 of the SIBO diet, eat smaller meals, ideally three to five hours apart. It's vital that you chew each bite thoroughly; remember digestion starts in the mouth! Drink plenty of fresh water throughout the day to stay properly hydrated. It's also important to manage stress during healing. Yoga, barre, tai chi, regular exercise and acupuncture can help reduce stress levels and keep you motivated to stay on track with the SIBO diet.

When treating SIBO symptoms, it's important to give your body time to repair while fighting the bacterial overgrowth in your small intestine. By eliminating FODMAPS from your diet for two weeks, and then transitioning to the GAPS diet and protocol, you can start the healing process and be well on your way to killing the bacteria causing your SIBO symptoms.

The SIBO Specific Diet

What is the SIBO Specific Diet

It is a combination of the Specific Carbohydrate Diet otherwise known as SCD, and Low FODMAP'S diet. SCD was developed by Elaine Gottschall, a biochemist and a biologist who wrote the book "Breaking the Viscous Cycle". She developed the diet for treatment of Crohn's disease, ulcerative colitis, celiac disease, diverticulitis, cystic fibrosis and chronic diarrhea. FODMAP stands for Fermentable, Oligo-, Di-, Mono-saccharides And Polyols. This diet was developed by Gibbson and Sheppard at Monash University for treatment of Irritable Bowel Syndrome.

Why use the SIBO Specific Diet?

There are several diets being recommended to treat SIBO.

The SIBO Specific Diet is great for those who have difficult cases of SIBO where other diets are not sufficiently providing symptomatic relief. Unlike other diets such as Specific Carbohydrate Diet (SCD) and FODMAPs Diet, Cedar Sinai Diet and GAPs the SIBO Specific Diet is the only one that has been specifically formulated to treat SIBO by leading expert in SIBO, Dr. Allison Siebecker. The SIBO diet essentially combines the SCD and FODMAPs diets.

Who can benefit from the SIBO Specific Diet?

The SIBO Specific Diet is a treatment for:Irritable Bowel Syndrome

- Irritable Bowel Disease- Crohn's disease, Ulcerative colitis
- Celiac's disease
- Diverticulitis
- Cystic fibrosis
- Chronic diarrhea or chronic constipation

Even if you've not been diagnosed with SIBO or any other gastrointestinal condition you can still enjoy this diet for its benefits in weight loss and increased energy.

How the Diet works

The rationale behind using the SIBO Specific Food Guide is to avoid foods that feed the bacteria that have overgrown and eat foods that are easily digestible and break down quickly in your small intestine. Foods that feed the bacteria are those that are composed of short and long chain fibers, starch and sucralose. Foods that are easily absorbable are simple sugars and have little fiber. This way the food you eat will be absorbed immediately so the bacteria don't have time to get to the food before you have utilized it.

Fiber is indigestible to humans, as we do not have the enzymes to break it down. We need bacteria to digest it for us because they do have the enzymes to break it down. Fiber is present in all plant foods but some more than others. The SIBO Specific Food Guide limits the amount of fiber you are consuming so as not to feed the bacteria.

Starch and the SIBO diet

Starch

Sucralose and the SIBO Diet

Sucralose

Foods that are fermentable such as artichokes, asparagus and grains stick around longer in your intestine and provide excellent food for bacteria. Foods in the SIBO Food

Chart (PDF) are classified into low, medium and high based on their fermentability. Generally you want to eat the "low" fermentability foods and restrict the "highly" fermentable foods. It has been found that having SIBO can cause lactose mal-absorption/intolerance as well as fructose mal-absorption /intolerance. Thus another element of the combo diet is removal of foods that contain lactose or high levels of fructose.

Below are general principles, helpful tips and resources for the combo diet. We know that if you are reading this blog it means you or someone you know is most likely in a good deal of discomfort and are ready to feel better. We want you to be successful. This information comes from personal experience, clinical experience and clinical trials. It is the best way we know at this time to treat SIBO. We know this diet involves making big life changes but it is worth it and it will help if done properly. Good luck!

Overview

The main principles of this diet are:

- No starch

- Low fiber
- Low fermentable fruits and veggies
- Watch portion size – this is based on fermentability of the foods
- No raw foods or beans at first
- Wait at least 4 hours between meals

What you can eat

As much as you want of: Any kind of meat

- Fat
- Lactose free dairy (examples below)
- Restricted and or tiered items: Download SIBO Food Chart here (PDF).
- Vegetables
- Fruit
- Nuts/seeds
- Squashes

What you can't eat

- No grain (yes, that includes quinoa and oats)

- No sugar
- No corn, soy or tubers
- No thickeners – carrageen, guar gum, agar
- No mucilaginous foods- flax, chia, seaweeds, licorice, aloe, astragalus, slippery elm
- No bone broths *(cartilage broth is not allowed but marrow both is allowed)
- No beans at first
- No garlic or onions

SIBO Food Chart

How to use the SIBO Food Chart:

When you first begin:

Eat anything from the “low” column

1 food/meal from the “moderate” column

Avoid the “high” & “SCD Illegal” columns

Do not eat raw foods or beans

The exception to these guidelines is if you know that you can tolerate something from the moderate or high columns. Then you can incorporate that food right away.

After you get the hang of it:

Try incorporating more of the moderate and even high column foods

Can start to eat raw foods and some beans

When to start:

If using as a stand alone treatment:

Start after SIBO breath test

If using as a preventative after antibiotic treatment (herbal or pharmaceutical):

Start diet slowly while on antibiotics so that by the time you have finished the antibiotic treatment you are fully on the diet. It takes a little while to get the hang of the new diet

Helpful tips

Incorporate Lactose free dairy

Ghee – great for cooking and baking

Aged Cheese – aged past 30 days

Dry Curd Cottage Cheese

24 hour yogurt – rich in probiotics, really helps to sooth stomach; is a helpful addition to diet for weight gain in the underweight

Bananas – can be really helpful especially with hydrogen type SIBO where you are having frequent diarrhea; use with caution if you have constipation as it may worsen symptoms

Wait at least 4 hours between meals – this is very important! You need time for your MMC to be able to clear out old food and bacteria

Wait at least 6-8 weeks before experimenting with foods that are "illegal." Trust us on this one, you don't want to have to start all over again. Your gut needs time to heal before you try foods that are more difficult to handle

Start the first two weeks of the diet with cooked foods only! This is important. Raw foods like salads are really much more difficult for your body to digest and can cause unwanted symptoms. After the initial 2 weeks it is usually OK to start eating raw foods again although in some it may take months so be patient

Don't over do it on nuts. There are a lot of great recipes for delicious baked items with almond flour. It is really easy to eat more than the diet allows and you will feel the consequences of this. Pace yourself with sweets

Add in new foods slowly. Don't experiment with multiple new foods at one time because then you will not know which is the one that has triggered you if you do end up having a reaction

Don't over eat acceptable foods; smaller portion sizes are easier to handle in the beginning

Weight loss prevention tips:

Eat lactose free dairy

Eat more food more often, set a timer if necessary

Try making shakes with yoghurt, nut butters, fruit and honey. My personal favourite shake is banana, honey, peanut butter, coconut oil and water or homemade almond milk

Add butter and coconut oil to your coffee in the mornings (We know it sounds weird but it is delicious and tastes like a frappé when blended)

Take digestive enzymes

Elemental Diet for SIBO

For a long time, researchers and clinicians treating individuals with gastrointestinal diseases believed that good therapeutic responses were only possible if the bowel was completely at rest. This meant that most patients were only able to gain necessary nutrients through intravenous feeding, which often meant longer hospital stays that still did not completely resolve these GI issues.

As a result, physicians began to investigate how a diet consisting of foods that were already in their "pre-digested" state may improve patient outcomes while also giving them a greater quality of life in the process. The elemental diet was originally developed in the 1970s for a couple reasons:

By a group of physicians investigating how breaking down certain proteins could improve both human and animal intestinal health.

1 For use in space exploration by astronauts on prolonged journeys where the problems of storage, ingestion, and waste disposal were important.

2 Basically, it has been shown that the elemental diet is one of the most effective treatment options for patients suffering from a variety of digestive conditions, particularly those struggling with small intestinal bacterial overgrowth (SIBO) symptoms.

In this chapther, we will detail everything you need to know about the elemental diet so that you can decide if this treatment approach is right for you. As you will see, using the elemental diet for SIBO treatment, inflammatory bowel disease, and other digestive issues is very effective.

What is an Elemental Diet?

Very simply, the elemental diet is a liquid formula (usually in powdered form) that contains all the essential nutrients humans need to live broken down into their simplest forms so they are easily absorbed.

Types of Nutrients Included:

Carbohydrates in the form of monosaccharides

Proteins in the form of amino acids

Fats in the form of fatty acids

Essential vitamins and minerals

By eliminating the need for the GI systems of these patients to perform normal digestive functions, as well as limiting the fuel source for bacteria, the elemental diet acts as a protective way to ensure that patients still consume all the necessary nutrients during this treatment period while allowing the bowels to rest and decreasing bacterial overgrowth. The main mechanisms by which the elemental diet helps a damaged GI system include:

1. Enable passive absorption of nutrients
2. Little to no stimulation of biliary and pancreatic secretions
3. Decreasing the activity of these enzymes prevents the ability of potentially painful endogenous (naturally occurring) agents present in the GI tract to release
4. Reduced load of potentially allergic components in food products
5. Improved nutrition consumption, particularly if a patient appears to be deficient in certain elements/vitamins
6. Reduce GI bacterial flora populations

Again, to achieve these physiological benefits, the main components of an elemental diet must include:

FATS – in the form of an oil (soybean, coconut, olive, etc.)

PROTEINS – in the amino acid form (or peptide chain form)

CARBOHYDRATES – NOT in the form of long chain and complex carbohydrates (dextrose, glucose and/or maltodextrin)

An elemental diet is recommended for individuals, typically with SIBO, IBS, IBD and other GI disorders, who experience the following symptoms:

Very high gas levels

Inflammation or a damaged gut

Methane positive breath test (this can be a more difficult type of IBS to treat)

Herbal medication sensitivity

Pharmaceutical medication sensitivity

Highly restricted diet

SIBO has appeared to be resistant to other treatments and/or antibiotics

Patient prefers a natural treatment option

Using the Elemental Diet for SIBO

As a result of an alteration in the type and/or number of bacteria present within the small intestine, patients with small intestinal bacterial overgrowth (SIBO) often experience a wide variety of GI symptoms including bloating, abdominal pain, diarrhea, constipation, gas, cramping and more.

As one of the most promising treatment options for patients with both moderate to severe SIBO, the elemental diet is a life-altering tool that has helped many patients reduce bacterial overgrowth and re-establish a more normal gut.

Compared to using antibiotics for SIBO treatment the elemental diet has been shown to be even more effective. Patients who were prescribed Xifaxan had a success rate of approximately 64%, while patients who underwent a 2-week elemental diet had a success rate of 80-85% in eradicating SIBO.

The success of the elemental diet for patients with SIBO is primarily attributed to the pre-digested state of the nutrients which are quickly absorbed, preventing the surplus of bacterial species from feeding on carbohydrates.

By starving bacteria in this area, an elemental diet is an effective tool in reducing bacterial overgrowth in the small bowel.

If using the elemental diet for SIBO, it's recommended that you use it for at least 2 weeks if not longer to see results. This allows the bowel rest and enough time to reduce bacterial overgrowth in the small intestine.

Full Elemental Diet vs. Semi-Elemental Diet

So what's the difference between a "full" elemental diet and a "semi" elemental diet?

In terms of the elemental product formulations, the main difference is usually in the protein structure. For example, a "full" elemental formula is usually just composed of free-form amino acids while a "semi" elemental formula has longer chains of amino acids or protein peptides like whey isolate. In terms of the elemental diet treatment process, a "half" elemental diet could also be when someone uses an elemental formula like Absorb Plus or Vivonex Plus and combines that with real foods using the elemental formula as a supplement for a certain amount of meals or extra nutrition.

Various scientific studies have found that patients with GI disorders show a beneficial response when their normal diet is supplemented with elemental formulations. In fact, these studies show that a full elemental diet may actually suppress the patient's diet and ultimately reduce their ability or interest in consuming normal foods following the completion of their elemental diet regimen. Overall, it has been shown that "semi" elemental diets are just as effective if not more effective in patients as compared to full elemental diets.

Studies Supporting the Full Elemental Diet

The elemental diet has become an increasingly popular treatment option recommended by physicians as clinical research has continued to demonstrate the efficacy of this treatment option for SIBO, as well as a variety of other GI disturbances. Below are some of these studies and the results of patients' health following completion of the "full" elemental diet.

PURPOSE OF STUDY

RESULTS

STUDY

Test changes in intestinal microbiota of Crohn's patients on the ED

Lower level of bacterial species present in fecal samples

Shiga et al. (2012)

Comparison of elemental and empiric elimination diets for the treatment of eosinophilic esophagitis (EoE) (chronic immune-mediated disorder of the esophagus)

Elemental diet with amino acid-based formula is most effective in maintaining remission of EoE; however, poor compliance rates are associated with elemental formulations that taste bad

Warners, et al. (2015)Markowitz et al. (2003)

Improving GI symptoms following radiation treatments for pelvic cancers

The different types of elemental formulations did not affect the patients' compliance in this study

Improved calorie and nutritional intake

McGough et al. (2006)

Both long term and short-term use of the elemental diet to manage Crohn's Disease

Severity of disease reduced

Reduces strictures, fistula and perianal disease rates in patients

Teahon et al. (1990)

Treatment of IBS/SIBO patients with abnormal lactulose breath test (LBT) rates

2-week elemental diet duration

Vivonex Plus used

Normalized LBT levels found in patients at both 15 and 21 days following when patients began the elemental diet

Improved bowel symptoms associated with improvcd breath test rates

Pimental et al. (2004)

Studies Supporting the Semi-Elemental Diet

It is important to note that the "full" elemental diet will only contain protein sources in their free amino acid form, carbohydrates in their simplest form of oligosaccharides or monosaccharides and fats as medium-chain triglycerides (MCT).

On the contrary, the semi-elemental diet instead can contain protein in the form of peptides of varying chain length, carbohydrates in the form of simple sugars, glucose polymers and/or starch and fats as MCTs. One of the biggest advantages associated with the semi-elemental diet in comparison to the full elemental diet is attributed to the different protein forms used in these two diets. While the free amino acid forms used in the full elemental diet prevent the patient from experiencing any type of allergic reaction to the protein component of the formulation, this form of protein does not prove to be effective in improving weight gain and/or malnutrition issues.

In fact, research has shown that free form amino acids cannot help build muscle for patients unless they piggyback on a dipeptide (or higher) protein bond 6, such as that which can be found when consuming whey isolate, for example.

Basically, a high-quality semi-elemental diet formula or semi-elemental diet that includes a little bit of food can be even better than a full elemental formula.

PURPOSE OF STUDY

RESULTS

STUDY

Compare a full elemental diet (enteral feeding) with a semi-elemental diet (amino acid-based feed combined with a whole protein-based diet) in Crohn's patients

Similar benefits were shown for patients on the full elemental diet as compared to those on the semi-elemental diet

Serum C reactive protein concentration levels were improved in patients on both diet regimens

Conclusion: Semi-elemental diets can be just as effective in treating Crohn's patients as elemental diets

Raouf et al. (1991)

Investigate the nutritional and health benefits associated with a semi-elemental diet

Semi-elemental diet has proven beneficial for patients in "high-risk" categories, such as those with Crohn's disease, short bowel syndrome, etc.

Semi-elemental diet has proven to perform just as well or better than full elemental diets in terms of tolerance, digestion and nutrient assimilation for patients with a wide variety of disease conditions

Alexander et al. (2016)

Investigate how a semi-elemental diet vs. a full elemental diet (using Vivonex-TEN) improves outcomes of adults with moderate to severe active Crohn's Disease

Greater remission rates after 1 year in patients on a semi-elemental diet as compared to a full elemental diet

Increase weight gain after 1 year in patients on a semi-elemental diet as compared to a full elemental diet

Royall et al. (1994)

Expert Advice Using The Elemental Diet

I had a chance to sit down with Jini Patel to discuss the elemental diet and her experience working with people around the world to heal their guts naturally.

Pros and Cons of the Elemental Diet So, you're thinking of using the elemental diet for SIBO or another gut illness. These are the pros and cons you should consider.

Pros:

- 80-84% success rate
- Easy to order formulations online
- Can dramatically reduce gas levels and symptoms in a 2-3 week course
- Can reduce the need for antibiotics and their side effects
- Allows the patient to take a break from preparing meals

Cons:

- Products can be expensive as the treatment course continues
- Not allowed to eat food for 14 days
- Die-Off Symptoms can be severe
- Some people don't like the taste

When is the Elemental Diet Recommended?

A physician may recommend an elemental diet for a variety of medical purposes, some of which include:

- Postoperative Management
- Nutritional support
- Particularly useful in healing patients following colonic and rectal surgeries, as well as neonatal and pediatric surgeries where adequate nutrition may be difficult to achieve following surgery
- Preoperative preparation
- Management of GI fistulae following procedures
- Associated with reducing mortality rates
- Balances nitrogen, potassium and magnesium levels in patients while on the diet
- Improved serum protein levels
- Management of malabsorption and maldigestion states
- Short bowel syndrome management
- IBD/IBS-SIBO
- Improved symptoms
- Reduced diarrhea, constipation, gas, bloating
- Nutritional management during cancer treatments
- Protection against weight loss
- Reduced rectal lesions during chemotherapy

- Protects against radiation damage that can affect small intestinal mucosa
- Liver disease and failure 7

When is the Elemental Diet Not Recommended?

- History of eating disorders
- Low body mass index (BMI), underweight patients
- Note that the elemental diet has been associated with increased body weight for individuals with malabsorption issues so this may not be an issue
- Diabetic patients
- Higher sugar content of the elemental diet
- Intestinal fungal overgrowth
- Can be used for these individuals if they are also prescribed an antifungal agent

Potential Side Effects of the Elemental Diet

It's not uncommon for individuals on the elemental diet to experience a variety of side effects, mostly due to the ingredients in the formula or the “die-off” reaction to a changing microbial environment.

Some common symptoms that should not alarm an individual on the elemental diet include:

- Feelings of constipation
- May be a result of decreased bowel movement due to decreased fiber
- Does not necessarily mean it is abnormal
- Most nutrients are being completely absorbed before food enters the colon
- Can be treated with magnesium, suppositories, enemas, herbal laxatives, etc.
- Nausea
- Can occur if the elemental diet is ingested too quickly. Sip slowly
- Usually begins in the first few days
- Will typically resolve itself if the formula is diluted

- Can also occur if a patient is also taking vitamins/supplements when on the ED
- Diarrhea
- May be a result of an ingredient in the formula that the patient is sensitive to or a die-off reaction
- Recommended that patients increase water intake and relax
- Feeling lightheaded
- Symptom aggravation
- Abdominal cramps
- Body aches
- Fatigue
- Blood sugar dysregulation

Elemental Diet Dosage

One of the most important aspects of the elemental diet is ensuring that you are consuming a sufficient amount of calories each day throughout the duration of your elemental diet. This is particularly important for individuals who are interested in maintaining their weight during this time.

If you are using just elemental shakes on your diet then you need to make sure to get the recommended amount of calories for your body weight. Be sure to use an online nutrition calculator to figure out how many calories you need, then order the correct amount of product for the duration of your treatment.

Homemade Elemental Diet

A patient may be interested in creating their own elemental diet formulations for a variety of reasons. Some patients have found that a homemade elemental diet was better for them because they could customize the ingredients used and switch up the carbohydrate and fat ratios. You can also save a little bit of money taking the DIY route. But, this method usually takes more research, time, and commitment to figuring out the exact specifications.

Most often it's recommended that patients who have successfully completed the elemental diet slowly transition back to actual foods by beginning with broths and a low FODMAP diet over the course of a week.

Additionally, it may be beneficial to continue to supplement with elemental formulations during this transition period. It is also highly recommended, particularly for patients with SIBO, that immediately after completing the elemental diet that they begin to take a prokinetic supplement to help stimulate the migrating motor complex which helps prevent the re-growth of unwanted bacterial populations.

Conclusion

In conclusion, the elemental diet is a great way for patients struggling with GI issues, nutrient absorption or a wide variety of other health issues to absorb important nutrients through their diet! The benefits associated with both full elemental and semi-elemental diets are well documented. While there are some formulations such as Vivonex Plus, which are hard to tolerate, there are a couple other products available, such as Absorb Plus, that can help make this diet a little easier on your taste buds.

With over an 85% success rate, particularly in patients with SIBO, the elemental diet is a clearly valid and highly recommended treatment option that may help you. Still not sure which treatment is best for you? Learn more about the different treatment options for SIBO.

Low FODMAP Diet and SIBO

Common Risk Factors for SIBOFODMAPs are a type of fermentable carb common in the foods we eat. They act as necessary “food” for our gut bacteria, but can cause severe digestive problems in sensitive people. The process of identifying and removing problem FODMAPs from the diet is known as a low FODMAP diet, and is clinically proven to treat IBS . SIBO shares almost all the same symptoms as IBS. In fact, studies show that between 30-85% of patients with IBS also have SIBO.

Due to this strong overlap, researchers suspect a low FODMAP diet may be beneficial for SIBO patients too, as it would “starve” the problem bacteria in the small intestine. Unfortunately, there has not been much research in this area and the current evidence is not clear.

It seems the low FODMAP diet is incredibly helpful when starting off, but requires a bit more flexibility for SIBO when reintroducing fermentable carbs. Just make sure not to start a low FODMAP diet until you have finished your course of antibiotics. The “bad” bacteria need to be active for the antibiotics to work.

There’s also limited research on the long-term effects of a low FODMAP diet. Following such a strict regimen for a long period of time may lead to detrimental effects on the bacteria in the large intestine. Summary: A low FODMAP diet may help initially by “starving” the problem bacteria in the small intestine. But studies have not yet confirmed it as a reliable SIBO treatment.

SIBO and Probiotics

Sibo and probioticsProbiotics is the name given to bacteria we intentionally eat for health benefits. They are essentially the opposite of antibiotics. It seems counterintuitive to treat SIBO – bacterial overgrowth – with additional bacteria, but recent research has seen success using probiotics instead of antibiotics. One small study of 14 IBS patients with SIBO found that a daily probiotic drink altered fermentation patterns in the intestine, consistent with reducing SIBO.

Another early study found that 82% of patients receiving probiotics for 5 days reported improvements compared to only a 52% improvement in those receiving the antibiotic metronidazol. These findings are in line with previous animal studies that observed similar benefits of probiotics
.

To be fair, though, some research found no significant benefits. One clinical trial on children treated with omeprazole found that probiotics didn't help, at least not in preventing SIBO. Until we know more, probiotics are not recommended until after completing the antibiotic protocol and a low FODMAP diet.

You also want to be careful of the type of probiotics you are using. Avoid any product with added ingredients like maltodextrin, which can end up feeding the bad bacteria.

Summary: Early studies have found probiotic supplementation may help with SIBO treatment. Its effectiveness has not been proven in clinical trials, though, but it's a promising area. Consider using them only after you have completed antibiotic treatment and a low FODMAP diet.

The SIBO Diet

To get started ridding your small intestine of bacteria overgrowth, start with a FODMAP elimination diet for two weeks. What are FODMAPS? They're foods that aren't fully absorbed in the body and end up fermenting in the digestive tract. The fermentation actually feeds the bacteria, making it more difficult to fight SIBO and SIBO symptoms.

What is SIBO and How Does Dietary Treatment Work

Small intestine bacterial overgrowth occurs when too much bacteria accumulate in the small intestine. This bacterial overgrowth causes numerous different digestive symptoms such as gas, bloating, constipation, diarrhea, and more.

How Dietary Changes Can Help

Now that you understand what SIBO is, we can discuss how diet can help.All effective diets used for bacterial overgrowth reduce food sources for bacteria in the gut. Bacteria mainly feed on carbohydrates so each diet limits the number of fermentable carbohydrates. This helps reduce the number of bacteria by limiting their food supply which then reduces digestive symptoms.

A few things to keep in mind are:

The combination of bacterial species is unique in each individual so food tolerance will be different for each person

Changes in diet can change the fecal microbial footprint rapidly

There is no sound evidence-based dietary treatment for SIBO although some diets have more research than others

Each diet modifies specific carbohydrates

Fermentable carbohydrates are important for overall health so restrictive diets should only be used short term until you figure out what combination of carbohydrates you can tolerate

What Are the Main Goals of Diet for SIBO?

1. To decrease bacterial fermentation and increase nutrient absorption

We want our bodies to get as much nutrition from our food as possible and not the bacteria in the small bowel Some fermentation by bacteria is normal and healthy but excessive fermentation is not normal in the small intestine

2. To allow time between eating to give your migrating motor complex a chance to clean

Research has shown that a large majority of people with small intestine bacterial overgrowth have a decrease in cleansing waves which can be an underlying cause of bacterial overgrowth

With weak migrating motor complex waves, it is important to try and allow at least 4-5 hours between meals Night time is when you have the longest period of fasting so it can help not eating late

3. To eat a balanced whole food diet with as much diversity as you can tolerate

It is the healthiest to eat a balanced diet so that your body can get all essential nutrients

Stick to the least restrictive diet that helps manage symptoms effectively

In general eat less processed foods which can exacerbate symptoms

If you keep these goals in mind you will be able to figure out a custom dietary treatment plan that allows for digestive symptom reduction as well as overall health maintenance.

Low FODMAP Foods to Eat

FOOD TYPE LOW FODMAP FOODS

Meat, Poultry, Eggs, Fish Chicken, fish, eggs, pork, shellfish, turkey, beef, lamb, cold cuts

Dairy (low lactose) Lactose free dairy, half and half, lactose free cream cheese, lactose free cottage, cheddar, colby, parmesan, swiss, sorbet, lactose-free yogurt, coconut yogurt

Non-Dairy Alternatives Almond milk, rice milk, nuts, nut butters, seeds, hemp milk

Grains (wheat free) Wheat free grains and flours without a ton of fiber: bagels, breads, noodles, pasta, pretzels, waffles, tortillas, pancakes, quinoa, rice, cream of rice, cheerios, grits, oats, sourdough bread, soba noodles

Vegetables Cucumbers, carrots, celery, eggplant, lettuce, leafy greens, pumpkin, potatoes, squash, yams, tomatoes, zucchini, bamboo shoots, bell peppers, bok choy, bean sprouts, collards, spaghetti squash, olives, green beans, rutabaga, spinach, ginger root, radish, turnips, corn, mushrooms, kale

Fruits (limit to one serving) Bananas, berries, cantaloupe, grapes, honeydew, grapefruit, kiwi, lemon, lime, orange, pineapple, rhubarb, passion fruit, kiwifruit, dragon fruit, papaya, clementine

Beverages Water, small amounts of low FODMAP juice, coffee, tea, gin, vodka, wine, whiskey

Seasonings, condiments, spices Basil, cilantro, coriander, lemongrass, parsley, mint, sage, thyme, homemade broth, chives, flaxseed, margarine, mayonnaise, olive oil, pepper, salt, sugar, mustard, vinegar, balsamic vinegar, pure maple syrup, vanilla, dark chocolate

Desserts Any made from allowed foods

High FODMAP Foods to Limit

FOOD TYPE HIGH FODMAP FOODS

Meats, Poultry, Eggs, Fish Anything made with HFCS or high FODMAP ingredients such as sausage

Dairy Cottage cheese, ice cream, creamy sauce, milk, soft cheeses, sour cream, whipped cream, evaporated milk, yogurt, custard, buttermilk, kefir, gelato

Non-Dairy Alternatives Coconut cream, beans, hummus, pistachios, soy products, coconut milk, black eyed peas, fava beans, kidney beans

Grains Inulin, wheat, wheat flours, flour tortillas, rye, chicory root, barley, bran cereals, granola bars,wheat germ, semolina, spelt flour

Vegetables Artichokes, garlic, onion, onion and garlic powder, asparagus, beets, broccoli, brussel sprouts, cabbage, cauliflower, fennel, okra, snow peas, sun-dried tomatoes, mushrooms, dried beans, butter beans

Fruits Large amounts avocado, apples, apricots, dates, canned fruit, cherries, dried fruit, figs, guava, mango, nectarines, pears, peaches, persimmon, watermelon, plums, prunes, figs, grapefruit

Beverages High FODMAP fruit and vegetable juices, rum, anything with HFCS, milk

Seasonings HFCS, garlic, jams and jellies, onions, pickle, relish, artificial sweeteners like sorbitol, mannitol, isomalt, xylitol, agave, coconut

Desserts Any made with High FODMAP

FOOD TYPE ALLOWED NOT ALLOWED

Protein Beef, pork, chicken, fish, eggs, bacon, shellfish, lamb Any meats that are processed, canned, breaded or made with added starch

Dairy 24-hour fermented yogurt, natural cheeses like cheddar, Colby, gruyere, Havarti, dry curd cottage cheese, swiss, Milk, cottage cheese, chocolate, ice cream, cream, feta, mozzarella, ricotta, primost, gjetost, Neufchatel

Vegetables Any fresh or frozen non-starchy vegetables Potatoes, yams, parsnips, okra, chickpeas, bean sprouts, soybeans, mung beans, fava beans, garbanzo beans, barley, chicory root, pinto beans, yucca root, seaweed

Fruits Any fresh fruit Plantains, any that are dried with added starch or sugar

Grains No grains allowed All grains and flours are avoided on the SCD

Nuts All nuts, nut butters and nut flours are allowed

Beverages Fresh squeezed juices without added sugars, weak tea or coffee, almond milk, gin, scotch, whisky, vodka, dry wines, club soda Milk, sugary drinks, soymilk, instant coffee, concentrate juices, beer, brandy, port wines, sake, sherry

Condiments All spices and condiments without starch or sugar such as honey Spices and condiments with starch and sugars added

Desserts Desserts made with nut flour, honey, and acceptable fruits Desserts made with any starch that isn't allowed or sugar besides honey

Which Beverages Are Ok

So what's best to drink to avoid digestive issues? It's pretty simple. Stick to water, light teas, lactose-free milk, and the occasional glass of dry wine if you like to have a drink.

You're best to avoid sugary drinks, too much alcohol, dairy with lactose, too much caffeine in coffee, sodas with Splenda, and too much fructose in fruit juices. Some drinks like herbal teas can even be helpful for some people.

For example, peppermint, ginger, and fennel tea can help ease gas and bloating. You can see our gut-friendly tea guide for more information on helpful teas.

SIBO Diet Plan – Week 1

Pancetta-Wrapped Pork Tenderloin

I'm sharing this recipe from The SIBO Diet Plan as it makes a wonderful holiday entree topped with cranberry sauce or other sauce. It also makes an easy week night entree as it can be made in less than an hour.

Serves: 6

Prep Time 10 minutes/Cook Time: 40 minutes

Ingredients:

- 2 tablespoons chopped fresh rosemary

- 4 teaspoons dried herbes de Provence or Italian seasoning (without garlic)
- 2 teaspoons garlic oi
- 2 teaspoons extra virgin olive oil
- 2 (1 pound) pork tenderloins
- 8 ounces pancetta, prosciutto or bacon
- Salt
- Freshly Ground Pepper

Instructions:

1. Preheat the oven to 350.

2. In a small bowl, stir together the chopped rosemary, dried herbs, garlic oil and olive oil. With clean hands or a pastry brush, spread the oil mixture over the tenderloins.

3. Wrap the pancetta around the oiled tenderloins and secure it by tying kitchen twine around the meat or by using toothpicks at 1 to 3 inch intervals as needed. Place the wrapped tenderloins on a rimmed baking sheet. Bake for 30 minutes.

4. Turn the oven to broil and broil for 5 minutes, or until the top is crispy.

5. Let the tenderloins rest for 10 minutes. Slice thinly, sprinkle with salt and pepper and serve.

Apple Cider Vinegar Drink

This drink mixes honey and vinegar for a slightly sweet and tart drink. Apple cider vinegar has myriad uses including helping regulate blood sugar and increase satiety. Yield: Four one-cup drinks

Ingredients:

- 4 cups water
- 2 tablespoons apple cider vinegar
- 1/3 to ½ cup clover honey simple syrup (depending on desired sweetness)
- 1-2 cinnamon sticks (optional)

Instructions:

- Mix all ingredients in a pitcher or large Mason jar.

- Leave cinnamon sticks in the pitcher or jar to add a cinnamon flavor.
- Pour into a cup and enjoy with ice or on its own.
- Keeps in refrigerator for about two weeks.

Sauteed Radishes with Thyme

Radishes are typically eaten raw but they are quite delicious when sautéed with fresh herbs. Makes 2 servings

Ingredients:

- 2 cups bite size pieces of radish
- 2 teaspoons ghee, butter or coconut oil
- 1 teaspoon fresh thyme leaves
- Salt and pepper

Instructions:

1. Heat a medium skilled over medium high heat.
2. Place the ghee, butter or coconut oil in the pan and heat until almost sizzling.

3. Add the radishes, thyme leaves, salt and pepper to the fat and sauté for approximately 7 to 9 minutes or until the radishes begin to soften and brown.
4. Serve immediately.

Nutrient Dense Burgers

The combination of pork, grass-fed ground beef and liver make this burger super tasty and nutrient dense. If you don't tolerate or like pork, you can use 1 1/2 pounds ground beef or any other preferred ground meat. These burgers make great leftovers and can be served with grilled veggies or a small salad. Makes 5-8 hamburgers

Ingredients:

- 1/2 pound ground pork
- 1 pound organic grass-fed ground beef
- 1/4 pound organic beef or chicken liver, pureed
- 2 tablespoons chopped chives or green onions
- 1 tablespoon dried Italian herbs (without garlic) or 3 tablespoons fresh herbs

- 1/2 teaspoon salt
- 1 tablespoon avocado or coconut oil

Instructions:

1. If the liver is not already pureed, place it in a food processor and blend until it is liquified.
2. Thoroughly mix together all ingredients, except oil, in a large bowl.
3. Form patties by hand. Depending on the size, you should wind up with 5-8 patties.
4. Heat large skillet on medium high and then add oil.
5. When oil is hot, add four patties. Cook approximately 5 minutes per side, depending on desired doneness.
6. Start a second batch of patties after the first is done, adding more oil first as needed.
7. Serve with lettuce, pesto, bacon or whatever sounds delicious! Jasmine Lime Cooler

Green tea is full of antioxidants! This refreshing cooler is a great summer drink to have on hand and is very easy to make.

Ingredients:

- 5 cups cold jasmine green tea
- 1/2 cup clover honey simple syrup (clover honey is low FODMAP)
- 3 Tablespoons fresh lime juice

Instructions:

1) Add all ingredients to a pitcher and mix well.

2) Store in the refrigerator for up to a week.

SIBO Diet Plan – Week 2

Celeriac Fries Two Ways – with Zesty Dipping Sauce

Celery root can be hard to digest for some people so try smaller amounts first.

Ingredients:

For the Celeriac Fries:

- 2 large celery root, cut into matchsticks
- 2 tablespoons avocado oil, divided
- 2 teaspoons salt, divided
- ½ teaspoon black pepper
- 1 tablespoon fresh parsley, minced
- 1 tablespoon fresh basil, minced
- ½ teaspoon ground cumin

For the Zesty Dipping Sauce:

- ½ cup plain, unsweetened yogurt (either dairy or non-dairy would work)
- 2 tablespoons coconut milk
- 1 teaspoon apple cider vinegar
- 1 teaspoon lemon juice
- 1 teaspoon fresh chopped parsley
- 1 teaspoon fresh chopped dill or basil
- ¼ tsp sea salt
- Pinch black pepper

Instructions:

1. Preheat oven to 400 degrees.

2. Peel both celery roots with a heavy-duty vegetable peeler or knife, then cut into matchsticks.
3. Combine matchsticks from one celery root into a large bowl and toss with 1 tablespoon avocado oil, 1 teaspoon salt, and ½ teaspoon black pepper, then spread onto baking sheet.
4. Combine matchsticks from second celery root into the same bowl and toss with the remaining 1 tablespoon avocado oil, 1 teaspoon salt, 1 tablespoon fresh parsley and basil, and ½ teaspoon ground cumin, then spread onto another baking sheet.
5. Place both baking sheets into the oven and bake for 35 to 40 minutes, rotating halfway through.
6. While the fries are baking, combine all ingredients for the zesty dipping sauce into a small bowl and whisk to mix thoroughly, adding more coconut milk (or water) to thin if desired.
7. Once celery root fries have begun to get crispy and turn brown on the outside, remove them from the

oven and allow to cool for 5 minutes before serving.

8. Serve with dipping sauce on the side, and enjoy!

Tapenade

Tapenade is wonderful to have in your refrigerator to serve with crackers, vegetables or a topping for pork or chicken.

Ingredients:

- 1 12 oz jar kalamata olives
- 1 teaspoon anchovy paste
- 2 tablespoons capers
- 2 tablespoons garlic olive oil
- 1/2 teaspoon dried Italian herbs
- pinch cayenne pepper (optional)

Instructions:

1. Add all ingredients except garlic oil to a food processor.

2. Process until mixed and well chopped.

3. Add oil and process until well mixed and slightly chunky.

Probiotic Ranch Dressing

This healthy, probiotic-rich ranch dressing is made from 24 hour yogurt but is reminiscent of ranch from a bottle – in a good way! It's great with veggies, on salads or with chicken wings.

Ingredients:

- 1 cup 24 hour yogurt
- 1 Tablespoon garlic oil
- 1 tsp dried chives or 1 Tablespoon fresh chives
- 1 tsp dried parsley or 1 Tablespoon fresh parsley
- 1 tsp dried dill or 1 Tablespoon fresh dill
- 1/4 cup parmesan cheese (optional)
- 1/2 teaspoon salt
- Fresh ground pepper to taste

Instructions:

1. Mix all ingredients in a small bowl or glass tupperware.

2. Dressing will keep for about a week in the refrigerator – if you don't eat it all before then.

Butternut Squash Lasagna

Ingredients:

- 1/2 lb organic ground beef
- 1/2 lb organic ground pork or sausage
- 1 tablespoon garlic oil
- 1 15 oz can tomato sauce
- 1/4 c extra virgin olive oil
- 2 teaspoons Italian herbs
- Sea salt & pepper to taste
- 1 medium butternut squash
- 3 cups freshly grated white cheddar cheese (aged at least 30 days)

Instructions:

Heat oven to 400ºF. In a skillet, cook meat with garlic oil. Pour sauce, Italian herbs and salt and pepper over drained meat, bring to low boil and then simmer for 10 minutes.

Cut the top and ends of the squash off and peel it. Cut in half, width-wise and remove the seeds. Slice the squash into 1/2 inch uniform planks.

Using a rectangle pan, lightly cover the bottom of the dish with sauce to keep the squash from sticking to the pan. Add a layer of squash, trying not to overlap the pieces. Spoon on the meat sauce mixture for the next layer and then add 1/3 of cheese mixture. Repeat two more times, with the cheese on top.

Bake for 45 minutes until the lasagna has a slightly browned top. Allow the lasagna to rest for 10 minutes before cutting.

SIBO Diet Plan – Week 3

Chocolate Granola

Prep Time: 5 minutes/Cook Time: 30 minutes Serves: approximately 10 (1/2 cup servings)

I'll admit it, once I make a recipe once, I want to try to make 10 different versions of it. Just like when I taste a new food once, I want to go try it in five different places, tasting the nuances of how each person made it their own.

So when I made a pumpkin spice granola recipe a few weeks ago, I knew it wouldn't be the last granola recipe.

A couple nice things about granola:

1) You can add or remove things you do or don't tolerate. Say you can't do almonds – fine, just remove them and add more pecans or another nut.

2) It's breakfast cereal. If you've been working on healthier lifestyle or a SIBO diet, you've probably been avoiding breakfast cereal. Typical off the shelf breakfast cereals are pretty much all fortified carbs – about as far from whole foods as you can get. But with making your own granola, you can have a lower sugar breakfast cereal that is delicious. Ok, and this one has dark chocolate – kinda devilish. But if you don't do well with chocolate chips you can leave those out. For those with IBS or SIBO, start with smaller amounts because nuts, seeds and coconut can be hard to digest for some people.

Ingredients:

- 1 cup unsweetened large coconut flakes

- 1 cup raw slivered or chopped almonds
- 1 cup raw pecan pieces
- 1 cup raw walut pieces
- 1/2 cup raw pepitas
- 1/2 cup raw sunflower seeds
- 1/4 cup chia seeds (optional)
- 1/2 cup dried cranberries
- 1/2 teaspoon sea salt
- 2 tablespoons melted coconut oil
- 1/4 cup maple syrup
- 1/4 cup cocoa
- 1 teaspoon vanilla extract
- 1/2 cup dairy free chocolate chips

Instructions:

1. Preheat oven to 350.
2. Cover a baking sheet with parchment paper or aluminum foil

3. Place the coconut flakes, almonds, pecans, walnuts, pepitas, sunflower seeds, chia, cranberries, sea salt, coconut oil, maple syrup, cocoa and vanilla extract in a large bowl. Mix everything together well.
4. Spread evenly on the baking sheet.
5. Bake the granola for approximately 9 minutes.
6. Stir the nuts and then make sure they are evenly spread across the pan.
7. Bake for another 9 minutes.
8. Remove the granola from the oven and then let it cool for approximately 5 minutes on a wire rack.
9. Add the chocolate chips and stir them into the granola. As they melt they should spread out somewhat evenly.
10. Let granola fully cool and then serve immediately or store in a Mason jar or other airtight container. Keeps for approximately two weeks on the counter.

Minted Melon Salad

Ingredients:

- 1 ripe cantaloupe, cut into bite size pieces
- 20 mint leaves, cut into julienne strips
- ¼ cup diced cilantro
- ¼ teaspoon white pepper
- 3 tablespoons lime juice
- 1 tablespoon olive oil
- ½ cup aged (30 days or more) feta cheese (optional)

Instructions:

Mix cantaloupe, mint, basil, pepper, lime juice, and olive oil in a medium sized serving dish.

Top with feta cheese and serve immediately.

Strawberry Lemonade Popsicles

Popsicles are a delicious snack or dessert during the hot days of summer. Organic strawberries are recommended since conventional strawberries tend to have extremely high pesticide residue and are in the Dirty Dozen.

Ingredients:

- 2 fresh organic strawberries
- 1/3 cup fresh or frozen organic strawberries
- 1 cup water
- 1/3 cup clover honey simple syrup
- 1/3 cup lemon juice

Instructions:

Remove the stems from the two fresh strawberries, cut them in half and then cut them in thin slices. Divide the strawberry pieces evenly among the popsicle molds. Alternately, you can use small paper cups.

For the 1/3 cup, if strawberries are frozen, defrost them until they're soft. With a hand mixer, blend the strawberries until they are pureed and no larger pieces are visible.

Mix the strawberries, water, simple syrup, and lemon juice in a medium bowl or pitcher. Taste the mixture. Add more water if it's too sweet for your taste, or more lemon if you like a more sour taste. Pour the mixture into popsicle molds or small paper cups. Store in the freezer until frozen. If using small paper cups, place a popsicle stick in the middle of the cup when it begins to freeze but isn't solid.

Serve immediately when frozen or store for up to two weeks. If you have any leftover popsicle mix, enjoy it as a drink!

Chicken Salad

Chicken Salad A chicken salad is an easy thing to take for lunch. See what's available in the refrigerator and go from there. What you'll find below is not so much a recipe as it is a starting point. Try different combinations and get creative!

Ingredients:

- 1 cup leftover chicken, shredded or cut into chunks
- Salad dressing of your preference – this can any sort of dressing including olive oil and lemon juice, mayonnaise, rice wine vinegar and sesame oil,

probiotic ranch dressing or whatever else you have on hand

- Nuts or seeds
- Fruit such as pineapple, raspberries, blueberries
- Veggies such as shredded carrots, spinach, butter lettuce, radish, steamed broccoli
- Herbs such as mint or basil

Instructions:

All you need to do is mix everything together in a bowl and eat it.

If you're making a lunch or dinner to take with you, you can add everything to a mason jar, putting the dressing on the bottom and layering everything else, placing any lettuces or softer veggies or fruits near the top. When you're ready to eat, shake it up and enjoy!

Flavor combinations to add to chicken:

Almonds, raspberries, chopped mint leaves, ¼ stalk celery, lemon and olive oil

Orange or tangerine, 1/8 avocado, chives, almonds, spinach, sesame oil and rice wine vinegar

Caesar salad dressing, 1/8 avocado, sliced hard boiled egg, romaine lettuce, and parmesan cheese

Artichokes hearts (1/8 cup canned is low FODMAP), walnuts, sliced red bell pepper, shredded carrots, bacon, chopped basil, green olives and ranch dressing

Mayonnaise or 24 hour yogurt, curry powder, halved grapes, walnuts, and butter lettuce

Spinach pesto (thin with lemon juice and olive oil or yogurt), cherry tomatoes, bacon, and cucumber

SIBO Diet Plan – Week 4

Sweet & Salty Mixed Nuts

This recipe is from my 1st book, The SIBO Diet Plan, which features a meal plan and a variety of recipes for people on varying SIBO diets.

In the book, I recommend waiting at least until week 4 to add whole nuts into the diet as they are hard to digest for some people. That said, they are great to have around for snacks, to bring to a cocktail party or give as holiday gifts. Prep Time: 5 minutes/Cook Time: 20 minutes Makes 4 cups of nuts.

Ingredients:

- 4 cups raw nuts or seeds (any combination of almonds, macadamia nuts, walnuts, pecans, sunflower seeds, etc.)
- 3 tablespoons maple syrup
- 2 tablespoons extra-virgin olive oil, coconut oil, organic grass fed butter of ghee
- 2 tablespoons fresh rosemary, thyme, sage or a combination
- 1 teaspoon smoked paprika (optional)
- 2 teaspoons sea salt, plus more as needed
- 1/4 teaspoon freshly ground pepper

Instructions:

1. Preheat the oven to 350. Line a baking sheet with parchment paper or aluminum foil.

2. On the prepared sheet, mix the nuts, maple syrup, olive oil or other oil/fat, herbs, paprika (optional), and 2 teaspoons of salt and pepper.

3. Bake for 15 to 20 minutes, stirring twice during the baking time. Make sure the nuts are evenly distributed on the baking sheet after stirring.

4. Remove the nuts from the oven and set on a wire rack to cool.

5. Taste and season with additional salt as desired.

Pumpkin Spice Granola

Serves: 10 (1/2 cup serving) Prep Time: 5 minutes/Cook Time: 20 minutes

This granola is for people that do well with nuts – because that's most of what it is. So if you're just starting a SIBO diet, start with small portions and see what type of reaction you have. If you know you're fine with nuts then enjoy this fall and winter spiced granola over yogurt, a smoothie bowl or for a morning breakfast cereal with your choice of SIBO friendly milk.

Ingredients:

- 1 cup unsweetened large coconut flakes.
- 1 cup raw slivered almonds
- 1 cup raw pecan pieces
- 1 cup raw walnut pieces
- 1 cup raw pepitas
- 1/4 cup chia seeds (optional)
- 1/2 cup dried cranberries
- 1 tablespoon pumpkin pie spice
- ½ teaspoon sea salt
- 2 tablespoons olive oil or melted coconut oil
- ¼ cup maple syrup
- 1 teaspoon vanilla

Instructions:

1. Preheat oven to 350.

2. Place the coconut flakes, almonds, pecans, walnuts, pepitas, chia seeds and dried cranberries on a baking sheet covered with parchment paper or aluminum foil.
3. In a small bowl, mix the pumpkin pie spice, sea salt, oil, maple syrup and vanilla.
4. Pour the spice mixture over the nuts and stir thoroughly until all nuts are coated.
5. Spread the nuts out on the sheet evenly.
6. Bake the nuts for approximately 9 minutes.
7. Stir the nuts and then make sure they are spread evenly on pan.
8. Bake for another 9 minutes.
9. Remove pan from the oven and let cool completely on a wire rack.
10. Store in a Mason jar or other airtight container. Keeps for approximately two weeks on the counter.

Sautéed Banana with Ganache

I stumbled upon this idea when talking with a client about the sautéed banana in my book (pg 171, The SIBO Diet Plan). Since I knew she was ok with a little bit of dark chocolate (as many people are, except those with histamine intolerance), I said, "Oh, and you can even shave some dark chocolate on top". But ganache, which is a sauce traditionally made with chocolate and cream, is even better. In this low FODMAP ganache, we substitute cream with any type of milk you prefer. A note on bananas: Ripe bananas are high FODMAP (high FOS in particular) but some people do really well with them. Unripe bananas are low FODMAP but tend to have resistant starch. So it's most helpful to try them in a small amount and see what works for you. Serves: 2

PREP TIME: 5 minutes

COOK TIME: 5 minutes

Ingredients:

- 2 tablespoons dark chocolate chips

- 1 tablespoon cream, coconut milk or other milk of choice
- 2 bananas, sliced
- 2 teaspoon honey
- 2 teaspoons butter, ghee or other preferred oil/fat

Instructions: Place the chocolate chips and the milk of choice in a small microwave safe bowl. Heat it in the microwave for 30 seconds and whisk it until the milk and chocolate are incorporated. When whisked, it should form a smooth chocolate liquid. If the chocolate doesn't completely melt, microwave it for 10 more seconds and whisk again. Heat a small sauce pan on medium high. Place the butter, ghee or other oil and the honey in the pan and let it melt. After it melts, add the banana slices and stir and saute the banana slices for approximately 2 minutes. Remove the banana and honey butter sauce from the pan and spoon onto two small plates. Pour chocolate ganache over the banana and serve immediately.

Steamed Broccoli with Lemon & Garlic

Broccoli, like other cruciferous vegetables, can be hard to tolerate for some people with SIBO. If you know you tolerate broccoli well, you can certainly add it to your diet earlier. Lemon juice is a “histamine liberator” but it is tolerated by many people.

Serves: 4

Prep Time: 10 minutes Cook Time: 10 minutes

Ingredients:

- 3 cups broccoli heads (no stalks)
- 2 teaspoons fresh lemon juice
- 2 tablespoons garlic oil or olive oil
- Sea salt
- Pepper

Instructions:

1. Steam broccoli for five or more minutes until soft but not mushy.

2. Place broccoli in a water bath with ice cubes and fresh water to stop the cooking process.
3. After several minutes, drain the broccoli and dry it with a paper towel so most of the water is gone.
4. Mix the broccoli heads with the lemon juice and garlic oil (or olive oil if you don't like garlic oil).
5. Season to taste with salt and pepper.
6. Serve immediately or chill.

SIBO Diet Plan – Calming Menu

Fourth of July Recipe Roundup!

Independence day is fast approaching and that typically translates to BBQs and picnics. If, "what should I make?" comes to mind next, here are some recipes to get you through the holiday.

Drinks

I adore sipping on this Jasmine Lime Cooler on a hot day. Or a Summer Punch is always refreshing. Lavender

Lemonade gives an old favorite a new twist. If you're worried about overheating, an homemade electrolyte drink (page 177 in The SIBO Diet Plan) will keep you hydrated during the day's festivities.

Mains

How can it be the 4th without Burgers?! The secret ingredient in these hamburgers is liver, a nutrient dense high protein food. Or maybe you're more of a turkey burger kind of person? And why not your burgers with a homemade BBQ sauce? If you tolerate some spice, these King Prawns with Spicy Salsa might be calling your name! Or get creative and make up a new version of a chicken salad.

Sides

Minted melon salad is easy to make but the light dressing kicks it up a notch! This colorful Mediterranean Zucchini Salad won't wilt and the zucchini noodles are fun to make. The Orange & Olive Salad on page 99 in the SIBO Diet Plan combines sweet and savory along with a delicious mustard vinaigrette. If you’re in a rush, buy some cut up veggies and throw together this delicious Probiotic Ranch Dressing. Or buy some hard aged cheese, grapes and make these quick, savory Herb Crackers.

Desserts

Chocolate chip cookies travel well and are everyone’s favorite. If you’re looking for something more patriotic, what’s not to love about Red, White & Blue Popsicles? These Strawberry Shortcake Cupcakes also look beautiful and delicious! And bars always satisfy – everyone will ask for the recipe for these nut butter blondies. Whatever you decide to make for your 4th of July I hope you have a fun, safe and satisfying holiday!

Low FODMAP Bone Broth Recipe

This recipe is adapted from Weston A. Price. Making bone broth with joints, chicken carcasses or other cartilaginous bones will result in a bone broth with GAGs (glucosaminoglycans) because the GAGs leach from the cartilage into the broth. GAGs are polysaccharides and while not high FODMAP, some people with IBS or SIBO will react negatively to them. It's important to test your individual reaction or simply make the bone broth without cartilage. The recipe below is for a low FODMAP bone broth, made without cartilaginous bones.

Makes approximately 16 one cup servings

Ingredients

- Approximately 3 pounds beef marrow bones
- Approximately 4 or more quarts cold water
- 1/2 cup apple cider vinegar
- 2 Tablespoons ghee or coconut oil
- 2 pounds beef stew meat
- 1 bunch green onions, green parts only, coarsely chopped
- 3 carrots, coarsely chopped
- 3 celery stalks, coarsely chopped
- Several sprigs of fresh thyme, tied together or 2 teaspoons dried thyme
- 1 teaspoon dried green peppercorns, crushed or freshly ground pepper (optional)

- 1 bunch parsley
- Sea salt to taste

Instructions

1. Place the marrow bones large soup pot with vinegar and cover with water and let stand for one hour.
2. Heat the ghee or oil in a large frying pan until hot. Add the stew meat and cook until well browned.
3. Add the meat and fat from frying to the soup pot as well as the green onions, carrots and celery.
4. Add additional water, if necessary, to cover the bones but make sure it doesn't reach the top of the soup pot.
5. Bring to a boil. With a wooden spoon, skim off and discard any scum that rises to the top.
6. Reduce heat to a simmer and add the thyme and crushed peppercorns or ground pepper.
7. Simmer stock for at least 12 and as long as 72 hours. Add water as needed to maintain the amount of beginning level.

8. Before finishing, add the parsley and simmer another 10 minutes.
9. Remove bones and stew meat from the pot with a slotted spoon. The leftover meat and bones will have less nutritional value but can be used as dog treats if desired.
10. Strain the stock into a large bowl or other container and cool in refrigerator.
11. When cool, remove any fat that has risen to the top.
12. Transfer to smaller mason jars or glass containers if desired and refrigerate and/or freeze. For refrigerated broth, consume within three days.